Aging Gracefully: A Pocket Guide for Middle-Aged and Older Adults

By
Andrew Harris

Aging Gracefully

Aging Gracefully: A Pocket Guide for Middle-Aged and Older Adults

ISBN: 9798397386463

Aging Gracefully

To my parents, who taught me the true meaning of aging gracefully through their strength, wisdom, and unwavering love. Your resilience and positive outlook on life have been an inspiration and a guiding light as I embarked on this journey to write this book.

To all who have shared their stories, struggles, and triumphs with me. Your experiences have shaped the pages of this guide, reminding us all of the incredible power within us to embrace aging with grace and dignity.

To my family, for their unwavering support, encouragement, and belief in my ability to make a difference. Thank you for standing by my side throughout the process of bringing this book to life.

And finally, to every reader who holds this book in their hands, may it serve as a source of empowerment, knowledge, and inspiration on your own path to aging gracefully. May it remind you that every stage of life is an opportunity for growth, joy, and fulfillment.

This book is dedicated to each and every one of you.

- Andrew

CONTENTS

1.

Introduction

Welcome to "Aging Gracefully: A Pocket Guide for Middle-Aged and Older Adults." This book is a compassionate and comprehensive resource designed to accompany you on the transformative journey of aging with grace, wisdom, and vitality. Whether you find yourself in the midst of middle age or are already embracing the golden years, this guide serves as a trusted companion, offering insights, guidance, and practical strategies to help you navigate the multifaceted aspects of aging and live a fulfilling life.

Aging is a natural and inevitable part of the human experience. It is a process that brings about profound changes in our bodies, minds, and lives as we transition through various stages of adulthood. Rather than viewing aging as a decline or limitation, we can reframe it as an opportunity for growth, self-discovery, and embracing the fullness of life. Aging gracefully is about approaching each passing year with resilience, gratitude, and a commitment to nurturing our well-being in all dimensions.

This pocket guide is rooted in the belief that aging gracefully is not solely determined by external factors but is deeply influenced by our inner attitudes, choices, and habits. It is a journey that encompasses physical health, mental and emotional well-being, social connections, purpose, and the ability to adapt to life's transitions. By intentionally cultivating positive habits and embracing the principles shared in this guide, you can unlock the potential for a fulfilling and joyful life as you age.

Throughout the pages of this guide, you will discover a wealth of knowledge, practical strategies, and empowering insights to support you on your unique path of aging gracefully. It is an invitation to explore new perspectives, challenge societal narratives about aging, and celebrate the wisdom and experiences accumulated throughout your life. This is not a one-size-fits-all approach, but rather a collection of tools and resources for you to tailor and adapt to your individual needs, desires, and circumstances.

As we embark on this transformative journey together, we will explore various themes, including the importance of embracing healthy aging, nurturing physical and mental well-being, fostering meaningful social connections, navigating life transitions, and finding purpose and fulfillment in the later years. Each section of this guide is carefully crafted to address the specific aspects of aging that have a profound impact on our overall quality of life.

Remember, aging is not a destination but an ongoing process, and it is never too late to embrace positive change and embark on a path of growth and self-improvement. This guide is not intended to be a quick fix or a definitive roadmap, but rather a source of inspiration, encouragement, and practical guidance to help you navigate the complexities and possibilities that come with aging.

Importance of embracing healthy aging

In this first section of our pocket guide, we will explore the profound significance of embracing healthy aging as a fundamental pillar for leading a vibrant and fulfilling life. Embracing healthy aging encompasses far more than simply managing physical health; it encompasses nurturing our entire being—body, mind, and spirit—to create a harmonious and balanced existence.

As we age, it becomes increasingly vital to prioritize our well-being and adopt healthy habits that promote longevity, vitality, and a sense of inner peace. Embracing healthy aging means recognizing the interconnectedness of our physical, mental, and emotional well-being and taking proactive steps to cultivate each aspect of our lives. It involves adopting a holistic approach that encompasses nutrition, exercise, stress management, emotional well-being, and cultivating a positive mindset.

When we embrace healthy aging, we empower ourselves to lead lives filled with purpose, joy, and vitality. It allows us to experience the full spectrum of what it means to be human, recognizing that our bodies, minds, and spirits are intricately intertwined. By nurturing our physical health, we can enhance our energy levels, maintain our mobility, and prevent or manage chronic diseases. By prioritizing our mental and emotional well-being, we can foster resilience, sharpen our cognitive abilities, and find fulfillment in the richness of our experiences.

Embracing healthy aging also involves cultivating self-compassion, practicing gratitude, and nurturing our social connections. It is about embracing change, finding meaning in life's transitions, and embracing the wisdom that comes with age. It is an invitation to honor the journey we have traveled and to celebrate the wisdom, resilience, and insights we have gained along the way.

Overview of the benefits of adopting positive habits

In this section of our pocket guide, we will embark on an exploration of the remarkable benefits that arise from adopting positive habits in the context of aging gracefully. Positive habits encompass the deliberate choices we make to enhance our physical, mental, and emotional well-being, nurturing a harmonious and purposeful life.

Aging Gracefully

By adopting positive habits, we unlock the potential for profound transformations in our lives. These habits contribute to our overall quality of life and empower us to experience the fullness of each passing year. They enable us to cultivate resilience, boost our physical vitality, enhance cognitive function, and foster emotional balance.

The benefits of adopting positive habits are wide-ranging and profound. Through regular exercise and physical activity, we strengthen our bodies, improve cardiovascular health, and maintain flexibility and mobility. Engaging in mental stimulation and cognitive exercises, such as learning new skills or pursuing creative outlets, supports brain health, memory, and overall cognitive function.

Positive habits also play a vital role in emotional well-being. By practicing stress management techniques, nurturing healthy coping mechanisms, and cultivating mindfulness, we can reduce stress levels, enhance emotional resilience, and find greater inner peace. Adopting positive habits related to nutrition and healthy eating can fuel our bodies with essential nutrients, support immune function, and reduce the risk of chronic diseases.

Furthermore, the adoption of positive habits extends to the realm of social connections and purpose. Maintaining an active social life, engaging in meaningful relationships, and contributing to our communities offer profound benefits, including increased happiness, a sense of belonging, and a deeper sense of purpose.

As we explore the benefits of adopting positive habits, it is essential to recognize that these habits are not one-size-fits-all. Each individual's journey is unique, and it is vital to listen to our bodies, honor our personal preferences, and adapt these habits to our specific circumstances and needs.

Throughout the pages of this guide, we will provide practical guidance, evidence-based insights, and actionable tips to help you incorporate positive habits into your daily life. We will explore various areas, such as nutrition, exercise, mindfulness practices, social engagement, and finding purpose, offering a comprehensive roadmap for embracing positive habits that contribute to aging gracefully.

So, let us embark together on this transformative journey of adopting positive habits. By embracing the power of intentional choices, nurturing our well-being, and fostering a renewed sense of purpose, we can embark on a remarkable chapter of our lives—a chapter filled with vitality, joy, and the embrace of the beauty and wisdom that come with aging gracefully.

2.

Healthy Aging Habits

Nutritional Guidelines for Aging Adults

In this chapter, we explore the importance of adopting healthy aging habits, with a particular focus on nutrition. As middle-aged and older adults, nourishing our bodies with a balanced diet becomes increasingly crucial for maintaining optimal health, vitality, and longevity. By following nutritional guidelines tailored to our unique needs, we can empower ourselves to age gracefully, enhance our well-being, and embrace a vibrant and fulfilling life.

Importance of a Balanced Diet

A balanced diet forms the cornerstone of healthy aging habits, providing our bodies with the necessary nutrients, energy, and resilience to thrive as we age. Embracing a balanced diet involves consuming a diverse array of food groups, each contributing to our overall health and well-being.

A balanced diet promotes moderation and incorporates whole, nutrient-dense foods while limiting the consumption of processed foods, refined sugars, and unhealthy fats. By adopting this approach, we support vital bodily functions, maintain a healthy weight, and reduce the risk of chronic conditions commonly associated with aging, such as cardiovascular disease, diabetes, and certain cancers. Furthermore, a balanced diet enhances cognitive function, promotes healthy digestion, and supports bone and muscle health.

Key Nutrients for Vitality and Longevity
Within a balanced diet, certain nutrients play a pivotal role in supporting healthy aging. As we age, our bodies may require adjustments in our nutrient intake to address changing metabolic processes and age-related changes. By focusing on key nutrients, we can optimize our nutritional status and promote vitality and longevity.

a. Protein: Adequate protein intake is essential for maintaining muscle mass, strength, and overall physical function. Aging adults should incorporate lean sources of protein, such as poultry, fish, legumes, and dairy products, into their diet. Protein facilitates muscle recovery, preserves bone health, and supports immune function, promoting healthy aging.

b. Fiber: Dietary fiber plays a crucial role in maintaining digestive health, managing weight, and reducing the risk of chronic diseases such as heart disease and diabetes. Whole grains, fruits, vegetables, and legumes are excellent sources of dietary fiber and should be incorporated into daily meals to support optimal well-being.

Fitness Routines for Maintaining Overall Health

In addition to nutrition, incorporating regular physical activity is paramount to healthy aging habits. Fitness routines tailored to middle-aged and older adults help maintain overall health, enhance cardiovascular fitness, and promote mobility and flexibility.

Aerobic Exercises for Cardiovascular Fitness

Engaging in aerobic exercises is vital for promoting cardiovascular health and maintaining optimal fitness levels. Activities such as brisk walking, cycling, swimming, or dancing help strengthen the heart, improve circulation, and boost endurance. Regular aerobic exercise also aids in weight management, reduces the risk of chronic conditions, and enhances overall well-being.

Strength and Flexibility Exercises for Maintaining Mobility

Strength and flexibility exercises play a pivotal role in maintaining mobility, preventing muscle loss, and promoting independence as we age. Incorporating resistance training using weights, resistance bands, or bodyweight exercises helps build and maintain muscle mass, improves bone density, and supports joint health. Flexibility exercises such as yoga or stretching routines enhance range of motion, reduce stiffness, and promote balance and coordination.

By incorporating a well-rounded fitness routine that combines aerobic exercises, strength training, and flexibility exercises, we can enhance our physical capabilities, support healthy aging, and improve overall quality of life. Regular physical activity not only contributes to physical well-being but also provides mental and emotional benefits, including stress reduction, improved mood, and increased cognitive function.

Strategies for Managing Stress and Promoting Emotional Well-being

Managing stress and promoting emotional well-being are essential components of healthy aging habits. As we navigate the complexities of life, incorporating effective strategies can help us maintain a positive mindset and cope with the challenges that come with aging.

Relaxation Techniques

Engaging in relaxation techniques can help reduce stress levels and promote a sense of calm. Practices such as deep breathing exercises, progressive muscle relaxation, and guided imagery can be incorporated into our daily routine to alleviate tension, improve sleep quality, and enhance overall well-being. Taking time for relaxation allows us to recharge and find balance in our lives.

Mindfulness and Meditation Practices

Mindfulness and meditation practices cultivate present-moment awareness and foster a deep connection with our thoughts, feelings, and surroundings. By incorporating mindfulness into our lives, we can develop resilience, improve concentration, and cultivate a sense of inner peace. Regular meditation practice has been shown to reduce stress, promote emotional stability, and enhance overall mental well-being.

By integrating stress management strategies into our daily lives, we can navigate the aging process with grace and resilience. These practices not only benefit our emotional well-being but also have a positive impact on our physical health, promoting healthy aging from the inside out.

Andrew Harris

3.

Maintaining an Active Social Life

Welcome to the chapter on "Maintaining an Active Social Life" in our pocket guide to aging gracefully. In this chapter, we will explore the importance of social connections and how they contribute to your overall well-being as you navigate the journey of aging. Staying socially engaged and fostering meaningful relationships can have a profound impact on your mental, emotional, and even physical health. By actively participating in social activities and nurturing connections with others, you can enhance your quality of life and age gracefully with a strong support network.

A. Benefits of social connections in aging

Research has consistently shown that maintaining an active social life is associated with numerous health benefits for older adults. Social connections provide a sense of belonging, purpose, and emotional support, which can help combat feelings of loneliness and isolation. Regular social interactions have been linked to improved cognitive function, reduced risk of mental health issues, and a higher overall life satisfaction. Engaging with others can also enhance physical health by encouraging healthier behaviors, providing motivation for exercise, and offering opportunities for shared activities and hobbies. The power of social connections should not be underestimated, as they play a vital role in promoting well-being and aging gracefully.

B. Strategies for building and nurturing relationships

1. Engaging in community activities and clubs

One effective way to maintain an active social life is by getting involved in community activities and joining clubs or organizations that align with your interests. This can include participating in volunteer work, attending cultural events, joining fitness or hobby groups, or taking part in local community initiatives. By immersing yourself in these activities, you can meet like-minded individuals, expand your social circle, and cultivate new friendships. Being part of a community provides a sense of belonging and offers opportunities for shared experiences and mutual support.

2. Utilizing technology for staying connected with loved ones

In today's digital age, technology offers various avenues for staying connected with loved ones, regardless of geographical distances. Embracing social media platforms, video calling apps, and online messaging services can help bridge the gap and maintain strong connections with family and friends.

Aging Gracefully

Virtual gatherings and online group activities allow for shared experiences, celebrations, and even support networks. Additionally, exploring online communities or forums centered around your interests can provide opportunities to engage with like-minded individuals and build new relationships. Technology can be a powerful tool for maintaining an active social life, particularly when face-to-face interactions are not feasible.

By actively seeking out social connections, engaging in community activities, and utilizing technology to stay connected, you can foster an active social life and enjoy the benefits that come with it. Remember, building and nurturing relationships requires effort and an open mindset. Embrace opportunities for connection, be willing to initiate conversations, and invest time and energy in maintaining meaningful connections. Aging gracefully is not just about physical well-being but also about cultivating a rich and fulfilling social life.

Andrew Harris

4.

Travel and Exploration: Adventures in Later Life

The golden years present a unique opportunity for middle-aged and older adults to indulge in the joy of travel and exploration. As we enter this phase of life, we have the freedom, time, and wisdom to embark on new adventures and create lasting memories. In this chapter, we will delve into the world of travel and explore the many ways in which we can make the most of our journeys in later life. Whether it's discovering new cultures, reconnecting with nature, or simply satisfying our wanderlust, travel opens up a world of possibilities for personal growth, enrichment, and enjoyment.

A. The joy of travel and exploration in the golden years

Traveling in later life is not just about visiting new places; it is about embracing the spirit of adventure, immersing ourselves in diverse cultures, and broadening our horizons. It provides an opportunity to break free from routine and embrace new experiences, fostering a sense of vitality and enthusiasm. Exploring unfamiliar landscapes, tasting exotic cuisines, and engaging in local traditions can ignite a renewed sense of wonder and discovery within us.

Furthermore, travel offers valuable opportunities for personal growth and self-reflection. It encourages us to step outside our comfort zones, face new challenges, and learn from different perspectives. By exposing ourselves to new environments and cultures, we develop a deeper understanding of the world and our place in it. Travel also promotes mental well-being by reducing stress, expanding our social networks, and stimulating cognitive function. The memories we create during our travels become cherished treasures that we can reflect upon and share with loved ones for years to come.

B. Tips for safe and enjoyable travel experiences
While travel is an exciting and rewarding endeavor, it is essential to prioritize our safety and well-being. By following a few simple tips, we can ensure that our adventures are not only enjoyable but also worry-free. Firstly, it is crucial to plan ahead and conduct thorough research before embarking on any journey. This includes learning about the destination, its culture, customs, and any potential health or safety considerations. Being well-informed allows us to make informed decisions and prepare adequately.

Additionally, taking care of our physical health is vital when traveling. This includes consulting with

Aging Gracefully

healthcare professionals, ensuring we have necessary medications, and obtaining appropriate travel insurance. Maintaining a healthy lifestyle through regular exercise, a balanced diet, and sufficient rest also contributes to our well-being during our travels. It is also important to be mindful of our limitations and pace ourselves, allowing for rest and relaxation as needed.

Another key aspect of safe travel is staying connected. Sharing our travel plans with loved ones and having a reliable means of communication can provide peace of mind for both ourselves and our families. Technology can be a valuable tool for staying connected, accessing essential information, and enhancing our travel experiences. From mobile apps to keep track of itineraries and bookings to online resources for reviews and recommendations, the digital age offers a wealth of resources at our fingertips.

5.

Fitness for Seniors

Welcome to the chapter on "Fitness for Seniors" in our comprehensive guide to aging gracefully. In this chapter, we will explore the vital role that physical activity plays in the lives of middle-aged and older adults. We will delve into the importance of staying active, the benefits it brings to overall health and well-being, and provide practical tips and tailored exercises specifically designed for seniors. By incorporating these fitness practices into your daily routine, you can enhance your physical capabilities, maintain muscle strength, improve cardiovascular health, and enjoy an active and fulfilling lifestyle.

A. Importance of physical activity for seniors

Engaging in regular physical activity is essential for seniors to maintain optimal health and age gracefully. Physical activity not only helps in managing weight and preventing chronic diseases but also boosts energy levels, enhances mental well-being, and improves overall quality of life. It is never too late to start or continue an exercise routine, and the benefits can be substantial.

Regular physical activity improves cardiovascular health by strengthening the heart and improving circulation. It reduces the risk of heart disease, stroke, and high blood pressure. Additionally, exercise aids in maintaining a healthy weight, which is crucial for reducing the risk of obesity-related conditions such as diabetes and joint problems. Physical activity also promotes mental well-being by reducing symptoms of anxiety and depression and improving cognitive function. It enhances mood, boosts self-confidence, and reduces stress levels.

B. Tailored exercises for seniors

1. Low-impact aerobic exercises

Low-impact aerobic exercises provide an excellent way for seniors to improve cardiovascular fitness without putting excessive strain on joints and muscles. Activities such as walking, swimming, cycling, and using elliptical machines offer cardiovascular benefits while minimizing the risk of injury. These exercises increase heart rate, improve lung capacity, and promote overall endurance. They are gentle on the joints and can be easily modified to accommodate different fitness levels.

2. Strength training exercises for maintaining muscle mass

Strength training exercises are crucial for seniors to preserve muscle mass, improve bone density, and maintain functional strength. Engaging in regular strength training helps counteract the natural decline in muscle mass that occurs with aging, ensuring that you maintain the ability to perform daily activities independently. Exercises using resistance bands, light weights, or bodyweight movements target major muscle groups and improve overall strength and balance. Strength training also supports joint stability and reduces the risk of falls.

Flexibility exercises for joint health

Flexibility exercises are essential for seniors to maintain joint mobility, prevent stiffness, and improve overall flexibility. Regular stretching exercises, yoga, and tai chi help to keep muscles and joints supple, increase range of motion, and enhance overall mobility. These exercises can also alleviate muscle tension, improve posture, and reduce the risk of injuries.

C. Tips for staying active throughout the day

1. Incorporating movement into daily routines

In addition to dedicated exercise sessions, it is important to incorporate movement into your daily routine. Simple activities like taking the stairs instead of the elevator, parking farther away from your destination to walk more, or doing household chores can contribute to increased physical activity levels. Set reminders to take short breaks from sitting and engage in light stretching or walking.

2. Engaging in recreational activities for fitness

Andrew Harris

Engaging in recreational activities not only provides an opportunity for fitness but also adds enjoyment to your exercise routine. Consider activities such as dancing, gardening, golfing, swimming, or joining a sports club. These activities promote social interaction, boost mood, and provide a fun way to stay active.

By adopting a holistic approach to fitness and incorporating a variety of exercises and activities into your routine, you can experience the numerous benefits of physical activity, improve your overall well-being, and age gracefully. Remember to consult with your healthcare provider before starting any new exercise program, especially if you have any underlying health conditions.

6.

Mental Wellness and Cognitive Fitness

Welcome to the chapter on "Mental Wellness and Cognitive Fitness" in our pocket guide to aging gracefully. In this chapter, we will explore strategies and practices that can help you maintain mental agility and promote emotional well-being as you navigate the journey of aging. The mind is a powerful tool, and by nurturing and engaging it, you can enhance your cognitive function, boost memory, and cultivate a positive mindset. By incorporating these practices into your daily routine, you can experience improved mental well-being and age gracefully with a sharp and vibrant mind.

A. Strategies for maintaining mental agility
1. Brain exercises and puzzles

Just as physical exercise keeps the body fit and healthy, engaging in brain exercises and puzzles helps keep the mind sharp and agile. Activities like crossword puzzles, Sudoku, word games, and brain teasers stimulate cognitive function, memory, and problem-solving skills. These exercises challenge the brain, promote neuroplasticity, and can even reduce the risk of cognitive decline and conditions such as Alzheimer's disease. By incorporating regular brain exercises into your routine, you can enhance your mental acuity and maintain cognitive vitality.

2. Memory enhancement techniques

Memory is an essential aspect of cognitive fitness, and there are various techniques and strategies that can help improve and maintain memory as you age. Practices such as mnemonics, visualization techniques, and association exercises can assist in retaining and recalling information. Creating routines, organizing information, and maintaining a mentally stimulating environment can also support memory function. Additionally, staying mentally active through lifelong learning, engaging in stimulating conversations, and pursuing hobbies that require mental focus can contribute to cognitive vitality.

B. Promoting emotional well-being
1. Coping with stress and anxiety

Managing stress and anxiety is crucial for maintaining emotional well-being. As we age, life transitions, health concerns, and other challenges may arise, affecting our mental state. Implementing stress reduction techniques such as deep breathing exercises, mindfulness, and relaxation practices can help alleviate stress and promote a sense of calm. Seeking support from friends, family, or professionals, and maintaining a positive outlook can also contribute to emotional resilience.

2. Cultivating positive relationships and social connections

Nurturing positive relationships and staying socially connected is vital for emotional well-being. Engaging in social activities, participating in community events, or joining clubs or groups that align with your interests can provide a sense of belonging and support. Regular interactions with loved ones, friends, and acquaintances help combat feelings of loneliness and isolation, boost mood, and enhance overall mental health. Building and maintaining strong social connections is an integral part of aging gracefully.

By incorporating strategies for maintaining mental agility and promoting emotional well-being into your lifestyle, you can foster a strong and resilient mind as you age. Remember, each person's journey is unique, and it's important to find what works best for you. Prioritize self-care, engage in stimulating mental activities, and cultivate positive relationships to support your mental well-being throughout the aging process.

7.

Healthy Eating for Longevity

Welcome to the chapter on "Healthy Eating for Longevity" in our pocket guide to aging gracefully. In this chapter, we will explore the importance of nutrition and how it can contribute to your overall health and well-being as you navigate the journey of aging. Adopting a balanced and nutrient-dense diet is a key component of healthy aging, providing your body with the essential nutrients it needs to thrive. By making informed food choices and incorporating nutritious meals into your daily routine, you can support optimal health, boost energy levels, and promote longevity.

A. Nutritional needs for older adults

As we age, our bodies undergo various changes, and our nutritional needs evolve. Understanding these needs is essential for ensuring we provide our bodies with the right fuel. Older adults often require fewer calories due to a decrease in metabolic rate, but the need for certain nutrients, such as calcium and vitamin D, may increase to maintain bone health. Additionally, maintaining a healthy weight becomes important for managing chronic conditions and reducing the risk of age-related diseases.

B. Designing a balanced and nutrient-dense diet

1. Importance of fruits, vegetables, and whole grains

Incorporating a variety of fruits, vegetables, and whole grains into your diet is crucial for obtaining essential vitamins, minerals, and fiber. These foods provide antioxidants that help protect against cellular damage, promote heart health, and support digestive function. Aim to fill half your plate with colorful fruits and vegetables, choosing a diverse range to ensure a wide array of nutrients. Whole grains such as quinoa, brown rice, and whole wheat bread provide fiber, which aids in digestion, helps maintain healthy blood sugar levels, and promotes satiety.

2. Managing portion sizes and mindful eating

Maintaining portion control and practicing mindful eating are key strategies for healthy eating. As we age, our bodies may require fewer calories, so it's important to be mindful of portion sizes to avoid overeating. Pay attention to hunger and fullness cues and eat slowly, savoring each bite. This allows for better digestion and helps prevent overeating. Being aware of the nutritional content of the foods you consume and practicing portion moderation can support weight management and overall health.

C. Recipes and meal planning ideas for healthy eating

1. Quick and easy nutritious meals

Preparing nutritious meals doesn't have to be time-consuming. Quick and easy options can be both delicious and packed with nutrients. Consider incorporating simple dishes like grilled chicken or fish with steamed vegetables, stir-fries with a variety of colorful vegetables and lean protein, or hearty salads with leafy greens, fruits, nuts, and seeds. These meals provide a balance of macronutrients and can be prepared in minimal time, making them ideal for busy lifestyles.

2. Snack options for sustained energy

Choosing healthy snacks is important for sustaining energy levels and preventing unhealthy food cravings. Opt for nutrient-dense options such as a handful of nuts, fresh fruit with nut butter, Greek yogurt with berries, or vegetable sticks with hummus. These snacks provide a combination of protein, healthy fats, and fiber, keeping you satisfied between meals and supporting overall nutrition goals.

By adopting a balanced and nutrient-dense diet, you can nourish your body, support healthy aging, and optimize your overall well-being. Making conscious food choices, practicing portion control, and incorporating nutritious meals and snacks into your daily routine will set the foundation for a long and vibrant life.

8.

Sleep and Aging: The Power of Restorative Rest

In this chapter, we delve into the significance of quality sleep for overall well-being, particularly as we age. Sleep plays a crucial role in promoting physical health, mental clarity, and emotional well-being. As we navigate the journey of aging gracefully, understanding the importance of restorative rest becomes essential for optimizing our health and vitality.

A. Understanding the importance of quality sleep for overall well-being

Quality sleep is not just about the number of hours we spend in bed but also the depth and restfulness of our sleep. As we age, our sleep patterns may naturally change, with a tendency to experience lighter and more fragmented sleep. However, this does not diminish the significance of sleep in maintaining our physical and mental health. Adequate sleep enhances our immune system, supports cognitive function, and helps regulate mood and emotions. It also contributes to healthy metabolism, weight management, and cardiovascular health. Recognizing the role of sleep in these areas empowers us to prioritize and optimize our sleep routines.

B. Establishing healthy sleep habits and improving sleep hygiene

To cultivate a restful and rejuvenating sleep routine, it is crucial to establish healthy sleep habits and improve sleep hygiene. One essential aspect of this is creating a relaxing bedtime routine. Engaging in activities that promote relaxation, such as reading a book, taking a warm bath, or practicing gentle stretching exercises, signals to our body that it's time to unwind and prepare for sleep. Avoiding stimulating activities, such as intense exercise or screen time, close to bedtime can also help facilitate a smoother transition into sleep.

Another important factor in improving sleep hygiene is creating a sleep-friendly environment. This includes making sure our bedroom is cool, quiet, and dark. Investing in a comfortable mattress and pillows that support our body's needs can significantly contribute to a more restful sleep experience. Additionally, addressing common sleep disorders, such as insomnia or sleep apnea, is crucial for enhancing sleep quality. Consulting with a healthcare professional to diagnose and manage any underlying sleep disorders can make a profound difference in our sleep and overall well-being.

Aging Gracefully

By understanding the importance of quality sleep and implementing healthy sleep habits, we can unlock the power of restorative rest and reap the numerous benefits it offers. In the following sections, we will explore strategies and techniques to create a relaxing bedtime routine and optimize our sleep environment, as well as discuss common sleep disorders and how to address them effectively.

Andrew Harris

9.

Aging in Place: Creating a Safe and Accessible Home Environment

Aging in place, the ability to live in one's own home and community comfortably and safely as we age, is a desire shared by many middle-aged and older adults. It provides a sense of familiarity, independence, and continuity in our lives. In this chapter, we will explore the benefits of aging in place and discuss practical tips for adapting our home environment to meet our changing needs as we navigate the journey of aging gracefully.

A. *The benefits of aging in place and maintaining independence*

Aging in place offers numerous advantages for middle-aged and older adults. It allows us to remain connected to our community, maintain social relationships, and preserve our sense of identity and belonging. By staying in our familiar surroundings, we can also retain a sense of control and autonomy over our lives. Being in a familiar environment promotes mental well-being and reduces stress, contributing to a higher quality of life. Moreover, aging in place often proves to be more cost-effective than relocating to assisted living facilities or nursing homes, allowing us to allocate resources to other aspects of our lives.

B. Tips for adapting the home environment to meet changing needs

As we age, it is essential to adapt our home environment to support our changing physical and cognitive abilities. One crucial aspect is ensuring proper lighting throughout the house. Adequate lighting reduces the risk of falls and improves visibility, especially in areas such as staircases, hallways, and entrances. Additionally, eliminating hazards, such as loose rugs or cluttered walkways, is vital for maintaining a safe home environment. Regular home assessments to identify potential risks and make necessary modifications can significantly contribute to our safety and well-being.

Installing grab bars in bathrooms and other areas prone to slips and falls is another effective way to enhance safety and accessibility. Grab bars provide support and stability, reducing the risk of accidents. Furthermore, exploring assistive devices and technologies can greatly enhance our ability to age in place. From mobility aids like walkers or wheelchairs to smart home devices that automate tasks and improve accessibility, there is a wide range of options available to help us maintain independence and safety in our homes.

By implementing these tips and making appropriate modifications, we can create a safe and accessible home environment that supports our evolving needs as we age. In the following sections, we will delve deeper into specific strategies and considerations for lighting, hazard elimination, grab bar installation, and the utilization of assistive devices and technologies.

10.

Managing Chronic Health Conditions

Welcome to the chapter on "Managing Chronic Health Conditions" in our pocket guide to aging gracefully. In this chapter, we will explore the importance of effectively managing chronic health conditions as you navigate the journey of aging. Chronic conditions such as diabetes, arthritis, cardiovascular diseases, and others can present unique challenges, but with proper management and lifestyle modifications, you can lead a fulfilling life and minimize the impact of these conditions. By understanding your health conditions, making necessary lifestyle adjustments, and maintaining open communication with healthcare providers, you can effectively manage chronic diseases and age gracefully with optimal health.

A. Understanding common chronic health conditions

Research has consistently shown that maintaining an active social life is associated with numerous health benefits for older adults. Social connections provide a sense of belonging, purpose, and emotional support, which can help combat feelings of loneliness and isolation. Regular social interactions have been linked to improved cognitive function, reduced risk of mental health issues, and a higher overall life satisfaction.

Engaging with others can also enhance physical health by encouraging healthier behaviors, providing motivation for exercise, and offering opportunities for shared activities and hobbies. The power of social connections should not be underestimated, as they play a vital role in promoting well-being and aging gracefully.

B. Lifestyle modifications for disease management

1. Diabetes management through diet and exercise

One effective way to maintain an active social life is by getting involved in community activities and joining clubs or organizations that align with your interests. This can include participating in volunteer work, attending cultural events, joining fitness or hobby groups, or taking part in local community initiatives. By immersing yourself in these activities, you can meet like-minded individuals, expand your social circle, and cultivate new friendships. Being part of a community provides a sense of belonging and offers opportunities for shared experiences and mutual support.

2. Techniques for arthritis pain relief and joint health

Arthritis, a common chronic condition, can cause pain, stiffness, and limited mobility. Incorporating gentle exercises, such as low-impact activities like swimming or walking, can help maintain joint flexibility and reduce pain. Additionally, applying hot or cold packs, using assistive devices, and practicing proper body mechanics can provide relief and support joint health. Working closely with a healthcare provider or physical therapist to develop an individualized exercise plan and exploring alternative therapies like acupuncture or massage may also be beneficial for managing arthritis symptoms.

C. Importance of regular medical check-ups and communication with healthcare providers

Regular medical check-ups and maintaining open communication with your healthcare providers are essential aspects of managing chronic health conditions. These check-ups allow for the monitoring of your condition, adjustment of treatment plans, and early detection of any potential complications. It is important to be proactive in discussing any concerns, symptoms, or changes in your health with your healthcare team. This open dialogue helps ensure that you receive appropriate medical advice, medication adjustments, and necessary lifestyle recommendations. Remember, you are an active participant in your healthcare journey, and effective communication with your healthcare providers plays a pivotal role in managing chronic conditions and optimizing your overall health.

By understanding common chronic health conditions, making necessary lifestyle modifications, and maintaining regular medical check-ups and communication with healthcare providers, you can effectively manage your health and promote well-being. Remember, managing chronic conditions requires a comprehensive approach that includes self-care, adherence to treatment plans, and ongoing collaboration with healthcare professionals. Aging gracefully is about empowering yourself to take control of your health and live life to the fullest.

11.

Embracing Life Transitions

Welcome to the chapter on "Embracing Life Transitions" in our pocket guide to aging gracefully. Life is full of transitions, and as middle-aged and older adults, you may find yourself facing various changes and adjustments. In this chapter, we will explore the importance of embracing life transitions and provide strategies to navigate these transitions with resilience and positivity. Whether it's coping with empty nesting, planning for retirement, dealing with loss and grief, or adapting to other significant life changes, this chapter aims to support you in embracing these transitions and finding new meaning and fulfillment in each stage of life.

A. Coping with empty nesting and transitioning into new roles

Empty nesting is a significant life transition that occurs when children leave the family home to pursue their own paths. While this transition can bring mixed emotions, it also opens up new opportunities for personal growth and rediscovery. Embracing this stage involves adjusting to a quieter home, reconnecting with your partner, or pursuing new hobbies and interests that were put on hold during the busy parenting years. It's important to remember that empty nesting is a natural part of the parenting journey and can provide an opportunity for self-reflection, personal development, and strengthening relationships.

Transitioning into new roles beyond parenting can be both exciting and challenging. It may involve redefining your identity and purpose. Exploring new passions, setting personal goals, and engaging in activities that bring joy and fulfillment can help you navigate this transition with grace. Embrace the freedom to explore new aspects of yourself and invest time and energy in self-care and personal growth. Remember, each stage of life offers unique opportunities for growth and fulfillment, and embracing empty nesting and transitioning into new roles can lead to a more enriched and purposeful life.

B. Retirement planning and finding purpose in post-work life

Retirement marks a significant life transition, as it represents a shift from a structured work life to a period of newfound freedom and leisure. However, retirement planning goes beyond financial considerations. It also involves preparing yourself mentally and emotionally for this new phase of life. Take the time to envision what retirement means to you and the activities and pursuits that will bring you joy and fulfillment. Consider volunteering, engaging in hobbies, or pursuing new learning opportunities to maintain a sense of purpose and fulfillment in post-work life.

Retirement can be an opportunity to explore your passions, spend quality time with loved ones, and engage in activities that you may not have had the time for previously. It's important to create a retirement plan that aligns with your personal values, desires, and financial circumstances. Seeking guidance from financial advisors and retirement planners can help ensure that you have a solid plan in place to support your lifestyle and goals. Remember, retirement is not the end, but rather a new chapter in your life journey, and finding purpose and fulfillment in this stage is essential for aging gracefully.

C. Strategies for dealing with loss and grief

As we age, we may encounter loss and experience grief in various forms, such as the loss of loved ones, declining health, or significant life changes. It's important to recognize that grief is a natural and individual process, and there is no right or wrong way to navigate it. Allow yourself time to grieve and process your emotions. Seek support from loved ones, friends, or support groups who can provide understanding and a safe space to share your feelings. Engaging in self-care practices, such as exercise, meditation, or journaling, can also help in the healing process.

Finding healthy ways to honor and remember those who have passed can bring solace and comfort. Consider creating rituals or participating in activities that celebrate their lives and preserve their memories. If necessary, seek professional support from therapists or grief counselors who can provide guidance and tools to navigate the grieving process. Remember, grief is a deeply personal experience, and it's essential to be patient and compassionate with yourself as you navigate through loss.

D. Navigating life changes with resilience and positivity

Life is filled with unexpected twists and turns, and learning to navigate these changes with resilience and positivity is key to aging gracefully. Embrace a growth mindset that allows you to view challenges as opportunities for growth and learning. Cultivate resilience by developing coping strategies, such as practicing self-care, seeking support from loved ones, and maintaining a positive outlook. Accept that change is a natural part of life and approach it with an open mind, embracing the possibilities it presents.

Maintaining a sense of gratitude and focusing on the present moment can also help foster positivity during life transitions. Reflect on the experiences and lessons learned throughout your life, and acknowledge your strengths and accomplishments. Embrace new beginnings with optimism, curiosity, and a willingness to adapt. Remember, you have the power to shape your own narrative and embrace life's transitions as opportunities for personal growth, self-discovery, and continued fulfillment.

12.

Living a Fulfilling Life: Pursuing Hobbies and Passions

A. The importance of pursuing hobbies and passions in later life

In this chapter, we delve into the importance of pursuing hobbies and passions in later life. As we age, it becomes even more vital to nurture our interests and engage in activities that bring us joy and fulfillment. Hobbies and passions not only provide a source of enjoyment but also contribute to our overall well-being, mental sharpness, and sense of purpose. They have the power to ignite our creativity, connect us with like-minded individuals, and unlock hidden talents we may not have realized we possessed. By exploring new interests and dedicating time to pursue hobbies, we embark on a journey of self-discovery and personal growth, enhancing the quality of our lives in remarkable ways.

B. Exploring new interests and discovering hidden talents

1. Engaging in creative pursuits such as painting, writing, or playing an instrument

Creativity knows no age limit, and engaging in creative activities can be incredibly rewarding in later life.

Whether it's painting vibrant landscapes, writing captivating stories, or playing a musical instrument, these artistic endeavors allow us to express ourselves and tap into our innermost thoughts and emotions. Engaging in creative pursuits not only offers a means of self-expression but also promotes mental well-being, stimulates cognitive function, and boosts self-confidence. It is never too late to pick up a paintbrush, start writing that novel, or learn to play an instrument. The journey itself is as valuable as the end result, and the act of creating becomes a source of joy and personal fulfillment.

2. Exploring physical activities like dancing, gardening, or hiking

Physical activities not only keep our bodies active and healthy but also provide a gateway to discovering new passions and interests. Dancing, for example, offers a joyful and expressive way to stay fit while immersing oneself in the rhythm and movement. Gardening allows us to connect with nature, nurture plants, and create beautiful outdoor spaces. Hiking opens doors to explore breathtaking landscapes and enjoy the benefits of fresh air and physical exertion. Engaging in physical hobbies not only promotes physical health but also enhances mental well-being by reducing stress, improving mood, and fostering a sense of accomplishment. These activities also offer opportunities for social engagement, whether through dance classes, community gardening projects, or joining hiking groups. The bonds formed and shared experiences with others who share similar interests can enrich our lives and provide a sense of belonging.

In conclusion, pursuing hobbies and passions in later life is an essential part of aging gracefully. It allows us to explore new interests, discover hidden talents, and experience a profound sense of joy and fulfillment. Engaging in creative pursuits and physical activities provides avenues for self-expression, personal growth, and social connection. Whether it's painting, writing, playing an instrument, dancing, gardening, or hiking, there is a world of possibilities waiting to be explored. So, let your curiosity guide you, embrace new experiences, and savor the journey as you pursue your hobbies and passions, creating a fulfilling and vibrant life that continues to blossom with each passing year.

13.

Conclusion

Congratulations on reaching the final chapter of "Aging Gracefully: A Pocket Guide for Middle-Aged and Older Adults." Throughout this guide, we have explored various aspects of aging gracefully, providing practical tips and valuable insights to support you on your journey towards a fulfilling and healthy life. In this concluding chapter, we will summarize the key takeaways, encourage you to start adopting healthy aging habits, and provide additional resources for further information and support. Remember, aging is a natural process, and by embracing it with intention and taking proactive steps, you can enhance your overall well-being and experience a vibrant and fulfilling life.

A. Summary of key takeaways

Reflecting on the information covered in this guide, it's important to highlight the key takeaways that will empower you to age gracefully. First and foremost, prioritize your physical and mental health by adopting healthy lifestyle habits. This includes engaging in regular physical activity, maintaining a balanced and nutritious diet, nurturing your social connections, and taking care of your emotional well-being. These habits serve as the foundation for a vibrant and fulfilling life.

Additionally, it's crucial to address chronic health conditions proactively and work closely with your healthcare providers to manage them effectively. By staying informed, seeking regular medical check-ups, and following recommended treatment plans, you can minimize the impact of these conditions on your daily life. Embrace life transitions with resilience and positivity, finding new purpose and joy in each phase of your journey. Finally, remember to prioritize self-care, practice self-compassion, and cultivate a positive mindset as you navigate the ups and downs of aging.

B. Encouragement to start adopting healthy aging habits

Now that you have gained valuable knowledge and insights from this pocket guide, it's time to take action and start implementing healthy aging habits into your daily life. Remember, it's never too late to make positive changes and reap the benefits of a healthy lifestyle. Start by setting achievable goals that align with your unique needs and preferences. Whether it's incorporating exercise into your routine, making mindful food choices, or dedicating time for self-care, every small step counts towards your overall well-being.

Seek support and accountability from loved ones or join community groups that share similar goals. Engaging in these activities collectively can provide motivation and encouragement along the way. Embrace the journey of adopting healthy aging habits with patience and self-compassion, understanding that it is a gradual process. Celebrate your progress, no matter how small, and stay committed to your well-being.

C. Resources for further information and support

To continue your journey towards aging gracefully, it's essential to have access to reliable resources and support. There are numerous organizations, websites, and books that offer valuable information and guidance on aging-related topics. Consider exploring reputable websites dedicated to health and wellness for older adults, such as the National Institute on Aging (NIA) and the American Association of Retired Persons (AARP). These resources provide a wealth of information on various aspects of aging, including physical health, mental well-being, financial planning, and social engagement.

Additionally, local community centers, senior centers, and healthcare facilities often offer programs and support groups tailored to the needs of older adults. These resources provide opportunities for social connection, education, and ongoing support on your aging journey. Don't hesitate to reach out to healthcare professionals, such as doctors, geriatric specialists, and therapists, who can offer personalized guidance and address any specific concerns you may have.

In conclusion, aging gracefully is a lifelong journey that requires proactive steps, self-care, and a positive mindset. By adopting healthy aging habits, nurturing social connections, prioritizing mental and emotional well-being, and embracing life transitions with resilience, you can enhance your quality of life and truly embrace the beauty of aging. Remember, you have the power to shape your own narrative and create a life filled with joy, fulfillment, and purpose.

Aging Gracefully